ADD (ATTENTION DEFICIT DISORDER): RECOGNIZING, COPING, AND HEALING ATTENTION DEFICIT DISORDER

A Holistic Approach To Treating The 7 Types Of ADHD

DR. BEENISH MASOOD

CONTENTS

Introduction

One of the misconceptions of parenting- among many others- is that parents feel their only responsibilities are feeding, clothing and educating their children. While these are indeed the very basic necessities of life, there is something else needed for living a fulfilling and complete life of quality, and that is developing their personality.

In order to nurture and develop your child's personality, you must first *understand* your child and his innate nature. Every child has unique and individual thought processes, experiences and approaches. Therefore, in order to help your child effectively you must *observe* and *scrutinize* him first. Observe your child while he's eating, playing or sleeping. Try and narrow down certain consistent or new behavior patterns and traits. What's his favorite game? What are his hobbies? Is he irritable? Does he adjust easily to new situations? Spend as much time with your child as possible. This will help you understand them better. You may even ask your child direct questions and cajole him to be frank with you. Analyzing these details will give you a good perspective of where your child stands and how you can help him overcome his weaknesses.

The reason why you must study your child's growth and learning is so that you can fully appreciate his physical, social, educational, cognitive and emotional abilities. Addressing these abilities will help your child excel in all walks of life and enable you to bring your child out of any behavioral disorder that he may be developing. As children are young, it is very easy to mold them and change their habits before they solidify into adulthood. Several studies have shown that children with behavioral disorders which persist into adulthood become a burden for not only themselves but also for people around them. They are unable to reach their full potential and are left behind other people their age.

This book will enlighten you about certain common behavioral abnormalities seen in children, especially Attention Deficit Hyperactive Disorder. It will also familiarize you with certain methods which you can use to treat your child.

CHILD DEVELOPMENT
THEORIES

❧

W hen talking about behavior, one needs to understand the dynamics of human behavior and psychology. The mind and the brain have finally been recognized as two different entities by scientists. They are closely intertwined yet; they develop independent of one another. While the brain is a functional organ with a specific structure and undergoes a series of consecutive changes during development, the mind is an intangible entity and has no specific pattern of development, which Is why it is a challenge to study about the mind.

Several psychologists have tried to theorize the development of the human mind, better referred to as human behavior. The have conducted a series of research trials and have studied children closely to come up with certain hypotheses. These child development theories have been broadly classified into:

- Psychoanalytic
- Cognitive
- Behavioral

- Social

PSYCHOANALYTIC CHLD DEVELOPMENT THEORIES

There are two prominent theorists who have used this approach towards child development. **Erik Erikson** proposed a theory of stage development and proposed that human growth continues to occur throughout one's entire life. According to him, each stage of development occurs in *response* to a difficult situation and is focused on overcoming that particular conflict. An example of this is when a child is reaches adolescence, the main conflict revolves around the establishment of a personal identity, perchance the adolescent fails to establish an identity, he becomes confused. Needless to say, the success or failure in overcoming a conflict in a particular stage affects the overall functioning.

The psychosocial stages proposed by Erikson include:

- Trust vs. Mistrust
- Autonomy vs. Shame and doubt
- Initiative vs. Guilt
- Industry vs. Inferiority
- Identity vs. confusion
- Intimacy vs. Isolation
- Generativity vs. Stagnation
- Integrity vs. Despair

Another theorist who has contributed to the psychoanalytic development of children is **Sigmund Freud**, the father of psychoanalysis. Freud always stressed upon the fact that childhood experiences mainly affected child development. However, Freud's theory is more about mental disorders.

According to Freud, child development is describes as a series of *psychosexual* stages, each of which involves the satisfaction of a sexual desire. If a child fails to complete one of these stages, then he becomes obsessed and fixated on that stage and this affects his adult life and personality. The five psycho-sexual stages proposed by Freud are:

- Oral
- Anal
- Phallic
- Latency
- Genital

COGNITIVE CHILD DEVELOPMENT THEORIES

According to these theories, children have a thought process which is very different from the thought process of adults. The most prominent theorist addressing cognitive development is **Jean Piaget**, a Swiss psychologist and educationist.

Piaget was one of the first psychologists to note that children are extremely curious about the world around them and hence actively try to gain knowledge. In fact, Piaget labelled children as 'little scientists' who were active in constructing their knowledge about the world. He thought that children's minds have a faster rate of processing knowledge and that's why they are so quick to learn everything. The stages of cognitive development proposed by Piaget include:

- The Sensorimotor Stage
- The Pre-operational Stage
- The Concrete Operational Stage

• The Formal Operational Stage

BEHAVIORAL   CHILD   DEVELOPMENT
THEORIES

The Behavioral aspect of child development has been most famous amongst theorists. A conglomerate series of facts have been derived from studies conducted by several theorists including **John B. Watson, Ivan Pavlov** and **B. F. Skinner**.

According to these theorists, who mainly study and observe behavior, development is in effect a *reaction* to rewards, punishments, stimuli and reinforcement. According to this theory, the child's thought processes and *mind* are not as important role players and *external experience*. According to these theories, experience is what makes a person's personality. One of the most renowned theories relating to the behavioral development of children is Classical Conditioning, proposed by Pavlov. Classical conditioning is a learning process which occurs when a child makes associations between an external stimulus and a stimulus which occurs naturally. Examples of this type of development include the response to fear or a frightening situation. Classical conditioning can be used to either develop a particular behavioral response or to get rid of a particular behavior.

SOCIAL CHILD DEVELOPMENT THEORIES

Social development has always been a favorite for psychologists. There are innumerable studies and theories on the social development of children. Prominent theorists in this category include **John Bowlby** who proposed one of the earliest theories of social development in children. According to Bowlby, the social behavior of children is determined by the early relationships that the child develops with his caregivers.

BOWLBY PROPOSED THE FAMOUS *ATTACHMENT THEORY* AND concluded that attachment is the most important component which aids in survival. According to Bowlby, there are mainly four aspects of a particular attachment. These are:

- Proximity Maintenance
- Safe Haven
- Secure Base
- Separation Distress

ANOTHER PROMINENT THEORIST WHO HAS WORKED ON THE social development of children is **Albert Bandura**. Bandura proposed that children learn new behaviors by observing other people. According to him, internal reinforcements such as a sense of achievement, pride and satisfaction are as important as external reinforcements in developing a child's personality. This is why children mimic the people in their immediate surroundings and learn most of their skills and behaviors from them. According to Bandura's social learning theory, the main aspects of the social aspect of learning include:

- Observational Learning
- Intrinsic Reinforcement
- The Modelling Process

1. Attention
2. Retention
3. Reproduction
4. Motivation

THE FINAL THEORIST FOR THE SOCIAL THEORY OF CHILD development is **Lev Vygotsky**, a Russian Psychologist, who lived through the Russian Revolution. Vygotsky suggested that the best mode of learning for children is by hands-on experience. He also suggested that parents, peers and caregivers were the ones responsible for the fine development of higher order functions.

An important concept to understand in Vygotsky's theory is the *Zone of Proximal Development*: this is the distance between actual development level of the child while solving problems independently and the potential development which occurs by solving a problem under either guidance of an adult or help of peers. In short, this refers to the skills and knowledge which the child is unable to grasp on his own but is able to learn with a little bit of help and guidance.

These are the main theories which affect child development. We have given a short introduction to these theories so as to familiarize you with your child's development and help you discover the cause of his particular behavioral disorder. The next chapter will give you a concise summary of some common behavioral disorders that children are dealing with today.

CHILDHOOD BEHAVIOUR DISORDERS

᚜᚛

Although episodes of bad behavior and temper tantrums are common to all children, there are times when these episodes become very frequent and tend to get out of hand; when your child is getting into trouble a little too often at school and he isn't getting along with other kids, then this is a sure-shot sign that your child needs your attention and help.

Children can develop a number of different emotional, mental and behavioral disorders as they go through childhood and adolescence. If these disorders are not given due importance, they will seriously affect your child's overall well-being and will persist into adulthood. Some of the more common and debilitating childhood behavioral disorders are described below.

ANXIETY DISORDERS

Although anxiety is a temporary phase that all adolescents go through, a child is said to have developed anxiety disorder when he suffers from extreme levels of fear, shyness and nervousness, to the extent that he avoids people and places. This is no doubt going to have an impact on the child's social skills. Anxiety disorders are currently amongst the most common childhood disorders. According to studies, children with untreated anxiety disorders tend to perform poorly in school.

Subtypes of anxiety disorders include:

GENERALIZED ANXIETY DISORDERS

The child is excessively worried about situations and has apprehensions which have no basis or relation to any past or recent experiences.

PHOBIAS

These are unrealistic fears that the child has of objects and situations.

PANIC DISORDERS

The child has bouts of 'panic attacks' which extend out to physical symptoms like palpitations, dizziness and sweating.

OBSESSIVE COMPULSIVE DISORDER

There is an overpowering need to perform certain actions or behaviors repeatedly because the child feels like he *has* to do a certain something one more time. For instance, examples include hand washing and counting.

POST-TRAUMATIC STRESS DISORDER

This disorder is a common sequel to distressing or disturbing situations such as war, natural disaster, a road traffic accident or a witness or victim of violence.

SEVERE DEPRESSION

Contrary to the previous belief that depression only occurs in adult life as a consequence of the stresses of daily, recently studies have proven that it can actually occur at any age and is quite common among children and is increasingly becoming more common, especially in adolescents. Around two out of hundred children and eight out of hundred adolescents are said to have major depression. Certain signs that lead to the diagnosis of depression are changes in:

1. Emotions: children cry for hours at end with no attributable cause.
2. Physical fitness: there is reduced appetite and sleep; the child may complain of pain or other vague symptoms.
3. Motivation: there is lack of confidence and motivation, as a result of which the child loses interest in daily activities and performs poorly in school.
4. Thinking process: the child becomes extremely and self-critical, he feels he is useless and incompetent.

BIPOLAR DISORDER

These disorders are suspected when the child exhibits excessive mood swings which alternate between an extreme high, which are said to hyper excited or manic phases, to extreme low moods of depression. Although certain periods of moderate moods seldom do occur in between these two extremes, they are still labelled as having bipolar disorder.

During the hyperexcited phase, the child usually talks excessively, sleeps very little or not at all and shows lack of proper judgment. Whilst at the other end of the spectrum, there is a bout of *severe* depression where the child may even border on suicide in extreme cases. The mood swings may occur throughout the child's life. This disorder has no definite treatment unfortunately; a combination of medicines is given so as to prevent extremes of both moods.

ATTENTION DEFICIT HYPERACTIVE DISORDER

This is a fairly common disorder and is recently being increasingly diagnosed amongst children and young adults. According to the latest statistics, this disorder occurs in five out of every hundred children. The affected child is fidgety and absolutely unable to stand still, tends to go round in circles and often keeps quiet. In order to definitely diagnose a child as having ADHD, the child must be seen to behave in this manner in a minimum of two different environments, such as school and home. There is further detail on the types, symptoms, diagnosis and treatment of ADHD later on in this book.

LEARNING DISORDERS

These are simply disorders related to difficulty in learning. The child is either unable to absorb the appropriate information or express it. The importance of identifying and treating learning disorders as soon as possible lies in the fact that these disorders impede the development of the child and manifest in later life as problems with self-control, attention, coordination, and written and spoken language.

CONDUCT DISORDER

Children affected with conduct disorders are basically rude and unmannered; they display extreme selfishness and show no concern for others. They also rend to repeatedly do the wrong thing like violating rules or other's rights. These children also tend to act out their feelings in a destructive manner. If left untreated, these children go on to commit more serious acts over the course of time. Children who *repeatedly* lie, steal, vandalize, set fires and are aggressive can be said to have a conduct disorder. This disorder is particularly common in adolescents.

EATING DISORDERS

These disorders are more common in girls as they tend to be more concerned with their looks and weight. These children are so afraid to gaining weight that they barely eat anything and starve themselves to bones, as in anorexia nervosa. Alternately, these children overeat or do binge eating and then go and vomit it out, as in bulimia nervosa. They may also take laxatives or enemas to quicken to the passage of food. They may also exercise excessively. These children are unable to maintain a healthy body weight and may end up having serious consequences related to malnutrition and starvation. Studies show that anorexia affects one in every hundred to two hundred adolescent girls each year, and bulimia affects one to three out of every hundred young girls each year.

AUTISM

This is a particular serious disorder where the children are said to have difficulty interacting with and communicating with other people. Autism manifests itself usually when the child is just one or two years old. They have an unusual and inappropriate behavior and tend to repeat certain actions over prolonged periods of time. Some children may even bang themselves on the head, rock to and fro or spin objects. The disease may be mild or very severe. It may also occur in combination with other mental disorders. Autistic children are unaware of other people around them.

SCHIZOPHRENIA

This is a very serious disorder in which the child may experience episodes of psychosis. When in these episodes, the child may have hallucinations, delusions and lose contact with reality. They withdraw from others and go into a shell of their own. Such children have very disordered thoughts and are unable to experience pleasure or any sort. They may sit in one place for hours at end without moving. Sometimes it becomes very difficult to diagnose schizophrenics because they may behave normally and keep their bizarre thoughts to themselves. There are effective medications which allay the symptoms of this crippling disease, however, the symptoms never disappear completely and may persist throughout life.

ATTENTION DEFICIT
HYPERACTIVE DISORDER (ADHD)

❧❧

W HAT IS ADHD?
As mentioned before, ADHD is a very important childhood behavior disorder and is increasing in incidence at an alarming rate. According to the CDC (Centre for Disease Control and Prevention), half of the children affected by ADHD are diagnosed by the age of six years. In the case of severe ADHD, children are diagnosed even earlier than the age of six.

WHAT ARE THE TYPES OF ADHD?

Attention Deficit Hyperactive Disorder is a neuro-behavioral disorder which affects nearly 5% of all children in America. It causes children to experience difficulty with self-esteem, self-control, attention and concentration. There are three subtypes of ADHD:

- ADHD, Predominantly Inattentive Type (also known as Attention Deficit Disorder, ADD)

- ADHD, Predominantly Hyperactive-Impulsive Type
- ADHD, Combined Type

WHAT IS ADD? HOW IS IT DIFFERENT FROM ADHD?

ADD is actually a subtype of ADHD. However, because the rate of incidence of both these disorders is on the rise and they both have certain obvious differences, they have been named and discussed slightly differently. These days the term, Predominantly Inattentive Type of ADHD is preferred over ADD.

Basically, both ADD and ADHD are brain disorders revolving around difficulty in staying focused on small every day activities like doing school work, brushing teeth and combing hair. The main difference between the two is that children with in ADHD, the child is excessively hyper and restless and the parent or teacher immediately suspects this disorder in the child, whereas in ADD, the children aren't as bursting with energy and restless and that's why they remain unnoticed for longer.

WHAT ARE THE SYMPTOMS OF ADHD AND ADD?

The symptoms seen in ADHD may include:

- Distractions and forgetfulness
- Switching from one activity to the other
- Difficulty in following directions
- Daydreaming
- Trouble with finishing tasks like homework
- Tendency to lose personal items like toys and books

- Fidgeting and squirming
- Incessant talking and interrupting others
- Running around constantly
- Touching everything they see
- Impatience
- Difficulty in controlling emotions
- Blurting out inappropriate comments

How is ADHD and ADD diagnosed?

The diagnostic criteria of ADHD, as specified in the 4th edition of the Diagnostic and Statistical Manual of Mental Disorders, divides the symptoms of ADHD into two categories, *symptoms of inattention* and *symptoms of hyperactivity and impulsivity.*

Symptoms of inattention

- Failure to pay attention to details and making careless mistakes in school work and other activities.
- Difficulty in maintaining focus on a particular activity or task
- Seems to be inattentive when being spoken to directly
- Failure to follow through with instructions and finish school work and other chores (*not* because of a deliberate rebelliousness or an inability to understand the instructions)
- Difficulty in organizing activities and tasks
- Avoiding getting engaged in activities which involve sustained mental exercise and focus
- Losing or misplacing items necessary for a particular task

- Easily being distracted by external stimuli

Symptoms of hyperactivity/ impulsivity:

- Fidgeting with hands and squirming in one's seat
- Leaving one's seat during class or other situations where leaving the seat is inappropriate
- Running around or climbing structures unnecessarily
- Difficulty in maintaining silence while playing an dengagign in toher activities
- Always on the go, as is one is 'running on a motor'
- Talking excessively
- Blurting out answers before completion of the question
- Difficulty in waiting for one's turn
- Interrupting or Intruding upon others conversations

When there are six or more inattentive symptoms, then the diagnosis is that of ADHD, Predominantly Inattentive Type. This is what is referred to as ADD.

The presence of six or more hyperactive/impulsive symptoms, then the diagnosis is of ADHD, Predominantly Hyperactive/Impulsive type.

When six or more of both types of symptoms are present, then the diagnosis of ADHD, Combined Type applies.

There are certain other criteria, which must be considered alongside the presence of the above mentioned symptoms, when diagnosing ADHD in children. These criteria are:

1. Some hyperactive or inattentive symptoms which cause disability must be present in the child before the age of seven years
2. The symptoms must be manifested in two completely different settings or situations
3. There should be clear evidence that clinically significant impairment occurs in social, academic and functional capacities
4. The symptoms do not occur during a phase of another co-existent psychiatric disorder such as schizophrenia or other psychotic disorders and cannot be accounted for by another mental disorder

When the diagnostic criteria mentioned above are used to classify a particular case of ADHD, you can be confident that your judgment is likely to be accurate.

ARE THERE ANY OTHER SUBTYPES OF ADHD? IF SO, HOW MANY?

According to ADHD expert Dr. Daniel G. Amen, there are seven types of ADHD, all of which revolve around three neurotransmitters present in the brain: *dopamine, serotonin* and *GABA*. According to Dr. Amen, not only do the seven types of ADHD have different symptoms, but they also have different treatments. The types are:

CLASSIC ADHD

This is characterized by easy distractibility, hyperactivity, impulsivity, disorganization and inattentiveness. Although the scans of the brains of these children appear to have normal activity at rest, there is significantly decreased activity seen in the prefrontal cortex (which is a part of the forebrain) during a task requiring concentration. This is thought to be because there is a decreased amount of blood flow to the prefrontal cortex, cerebellum and basal ganglia. The basal ganglia are involved in release of the neurotransmitter dopamine.

INATTENTIVE ADHD

This type of ADHD, similar to the previous one, involves low brain activity in the prefrontal cortex as well as low dopamine levels. It presents with a short span of attention, easy distractibility, disorganization and procrastination. The symptoms of hyper excitability and impulsivity are typically absent. Children affected by this type of ADHD are inherently introverted and have a tendency towards daydreaming. It is seen to occur more commonly in women.

OVER-FOCUSED ADHD

Children with this type show all the basic symptoms of ADHD, in addition to experiencing great difficulty in shifting their attention from one task to another. They simply cannot come out of a pattern of negative thoughts and behaviors. On scanning the brain of these children, an abnormally high amount of activity is found in the anterior cingulate gyrus, an area of the brain responsible for integrating activities and shifting concentration from one task to another. This is what makes it difficult to shift one's thoughts when doing different tasks. A deficiency of serotonin and dopamine is found throughout the brain.

TEMPORAL LOBE ADHD

This type of ADD has both core ADHD symptoms as well as temporal lobe symptoms. The temporal lobe is situated at both right and left sides of the brain. It is present just under the temple and mainly has the function of processing memory, moods and processing visual information receives from the nerves coming from the eyes. Due the area of brain involves, children affected by temporal lobe ADHD have problems in learning, memorizing and modulating their behavior. They tend to be aggressive, have a short temper, and may even be mildly paranoid. Brain activity is seen to be abnormal in the temporal lobe and decreased in the prefrontal cortex.

LIMBIC ADHD

This type of ADHD manifest as a combination of long term, subliminal sadness as well as the classic ADHD symptoms. Children affected are seen to be moody, lethargic, have feelings of guilt or hopelessness and have longstanding low self-esteem. This may be misinterpreted as depression, however it is very different. Brain scans show increased activity in the limbic portion of the brain and decreased activity in the prefrontal cortex at all times. The limbic part of the brain controls one's moods.

RING OF FIRE ADHD

Interestingly, this type ADHD doesn't show an underactive prefrontal cortex, rather, it shows increased activity *throughout* the brain. Due to this 'hyperactivity', the affected child is highly sensitive to touch, light and noise. The child shows episodes of unpredictable, nasty behavior, rapid talking, fear and anxiety. The name is attributed to the brain activity seen on scans, i.e. a ring of activity seems to surround the entire brain.

. . .

Anxious ADHD

Children affected by anxious ADHD have the typical ADHD symptoms and tend to be anxious and tensed at all times. Due to this constant stress, they experience physical symptoms of stress like headaches and abdominal cramps. These people always expect the worst outcomes and lose all judgment and cool in situations which making them anxious. They are very afraid of being 'judged' or being put on a spot. Brain scans reveal high levels of activity in the basal ganglia, producing excessive amounts of dopamine. This is what sets this subtype of ADHD apart from the others where low activity is seen in the basal ganglia.

As there are subtle differences in the different types of ADHD, it is understandable that the approach to each subtype and its treatment will vary from one another. These treatments, conventional as well as complementary, are mentioned in the upcoming chapters of this e-book.

TREATING ADHD

❧❦❧

There are innumerable medicines that have been introduced to curb and control behavioral and psychiatric problems. In fact, many more medicines are being developed as even more extensive research is being conducted. Conventional medicine has always been a savior for many patients, despite their side effects. It is backed up by scientific experiments and studies and the medicines are developed with immense precision and promise. Here, we have discussed methods to treat, or at the very least, alleviate certain symptoms of this disorder with and without medication.

CONVENTIONAL MEDICINE

The medicines which are currently being used for ADHD aim to restore the normal chemical balance of the brain by increasing or decreasing the necessary neurotransmitters in the brain. Doctors have proved the efficiency and effectiveness of these medicines by analyzing brain scans of patients before and after taking the medications. The scans after the medications were taken show that the brain activity has somewhat been restored to what is considered as *normal*.

The current treatment for ADHD, which is popular all around the world, is a branch of conventional medicine and is known as *Stimulant Treatment*. This type of treatment has proven to be effective in 92% of the patients with nearly 50-60% of them achieving complete remission!

The medications which are used for this treatment merely increase the *availability* of the concerned neurotransmitters to the synapses present between the brain cells. These neurotransmitters are responsible for carrying signals and information throughout the brain, hence their importance. The symptoms of ADHD manifest when these neurotransmitters become misbalanced and are unable to perform their intended function.

Contrary to the popular belief, medicines used to treat ADHD are *not* tranquilizers or sedatives; they improve the overall efficiency of different areas of the brain rather than slowing it down. Extensive studies have shown that the medicines being used to treat ADHD are extremely safe and effective. In fact, these studies have further gone on to prove that failure to treat this disorder with appropriate medicines results in the child resorting to other drugs for comfort; poor performance in school; low self-esteem; inability to cope with a variety of social situations and an over-reaction to changing or unfavorable circumstances. Undoubtedly, this leads to a disturbed and unsuccessful adult life. It has also been seen that failure to treat ADHD results in a decreased amount of white matter in the brains of these children. Having said this, in *all* cases, it is recommended that behavioral therapy be initiated first, before introducing medications into the treatment regime. Once the behavioral therapy has been initiated, medications should be introduced. According to research carried out in the State University of New York, the most effective way to improve the behavior of ADHD children is to combine medication with behavior modification therapy.

Certain medications with their generic and market names, and the FDA approved age groups in which they can be administered are mentioned below:

3 YEARS AND OLDER

- Adderall® (amphetamine)
- Dexedrine® (dextroamphetamine)
- **Vyvanse®** (lisdexamfetamine dimesylate)

6 YEARS AND OLDER

- Concerta® (methylphenidate)
- **Desoxyn®** (methamphetamine hydrochloride)
- **Focalin®** (dexmethylphenidate)
- **Metadate CD®** (methylphenidate)
- **Ritalin®** (methylphenidate)
- **Daytrana®** (methylphenidate)
- **Straterra®** (atomoxetine)

6 YEARS TO 17 YEARS

- **Intuniv®** (guanfacine, alpha-2-adrenergic agonist)

STIMULANT MEDICATIONS ARE SLIGHTLY DIFFERENT FROM

other medicines in that their doses are *not* dependent on the child's weight. Rather, clinicians must use increasing doses if they have to in order to achieve the desired results.

COMPLEMENTARY MEDICINE

Coming towards more natural methods of treatment, also known as complementary medicine, the reason one thinks twice before using conventional medication for ADHD, is that it is mainly a disease of children; it is never wise to expose growing children to synthetic compounds and medications just as it isn't wise for a pregnant woman to consume medications. The initial most and recommended first line treatment for ADHD and other behavioral disorders is behavioral therapies.

BEHAVIOR MODIFICATION THERAPY

As mentioned before, behavior modification therapy is the first and foremost treatment for children with ADHD. After having conducting several surveys and researches, renowned psychologist and professor of counseling, Gregory A. Fabiano, has devised certain behavior treatments which fall into three main categories:

PARENT PROGRAMS

These programs aim to teach parents certain strategies in order to help their children succeed. It encourages parents to *recognize their children's good behavior* rather than always pointing out their behavior on bad days. The parents are advised to praise the good or even normal behavior that these children manage to pull off and hence, reinforce this sort of behavior by appreciating them. Once these kids are given attention for their good behavior, they will be compelled to behave well in the future as well.

. . .

TEACHER PROGRAMS

The one person most influential in a child's life after his parents is his teacher. Teachers are advised to use certain behavioral strategies for the classroom, whereby they give *step by step, clear and concise instructions* to children and also *warn the children beforehand* of the consequences if they do not pay attention. Another tried and tested approach for teachers is *contingency management*; the children report cards *daily*, which have a summary of how well that child has behaved on that particular day, i.e. by doing their homework properly and waiting for their turn. Once the children have met these particular goals, they are awarded accordingly.

RECREATIONAL PROGRAMS

These programs are devised to enable children with ADHD to interact with others at places like summer camps. The activities lined up for kids here include sports, arts and crafts and other typical camping activities. This is a different and innovative therapy for children who are affected by ADHD. The sessions may extend up to several weeks. Children are taught to work in groups and co-operate with others. They are also taught how to use corporate management strategies in their play. Such therapies enable children to not only learn social skills, but also learn sports as well as develop a team spirit.

Behavioral therapies are advised to be started even before children start school. It is up to parents to get involved in their child's development.

LIFESTYLE CHANGES

Yes, it's *that* easy. Simply alter a few things in the child's daily routine and one will notice a definite change in his behavior!

One of the major changes one can make is by incorporating at least a few minutes of *physical activity* in the child's daily routine. Research has shown that just a few minutes of exercise is an effective method of stress release and helps children become more focused and perform better in school.

Another minor lifestyle change can be altering one's *sleeping pattern*. It has been proved by various studies that children can improve their behavior and avoid restlessness by simply sleeping an extra half hour. Alternately, lack of sleep serves as a fuel for emotional outbursts and temper tantrums.

OTHER NON-MEDICATION TREATMENTS FOR ADHD

Apart from these non-medication treatments, certain natural substances have been found to be very effective for children with ADHD. These substances include:

- **Protein**: Children who eat more protein show more improvement than those who don't. The child's diet should consist of a variety of protein including yoghurt, protein shakes, fish, eggs, legumes, fish, white meat and only moderate amounts of lean red meat.
- **Omega-3, fatty acids**: These are essential fatty acids which have found to be low in children affected by ADHD. Therefore, regular supplements of omega-3 fatty acids must be consumed by affected children. Foods rich in this essential fatty acid include walnuts, leafy greens, spinach, fish and flax seeds.

- **Iron**: Studies have shown that regular iron supplements were associated with lower levels of hyper activity in affected children.
- **French maritime bark**: This is a herb which was found to be associated with improved behavior and concentration in children specifically affected by ADD.

CERTAIN FOODS TO *AVOID* INCLUDE:

- **Artificial colors**: Artificial foods and colors are rich in natural salicylates. Symptoms of ADHD tend to improve when their consumption is limited. Natural salicylates are also present in several fruits.
- **Sugars**: This is a well-known 'culprit' amongst parents. Sugar is known to give children a sugar high and hence cause them to become hyper excited and restless. Needless to say, this food must be avoided by children affected by all types of ADHD.

HAVING EXPLORED ALL MODES OF TREATMENT, IT IS EASY TO deduce that perhaps the *most* effective treatment would be to include a bit of all types of treatments. Therefore, according to ADHD expert, Dr. Daniel G. Amen, a series of unique combination treatments are offered for each of the seven types of ADHD subtypes that he has described.

. . .

THE CLASSIFICATION OF ADHD INTO SEVEN TYPES IS BASED on the minor differences in the area of brain affected and the neurotransmitter which are in deficient or in excess. Consequently, the treatments of all seven types are different from one another. These treatments, according to the subtypes mentioned in the previous chapter, are given below:

- **Classic ADHD:**

DUE TO DEFICIENT DOPAMINE LEVELS, THE AIM HERE IS TOO increase dopamine levels and hence improve focus. This effect can be achieved by stimulating medicines such as Ritalin, Adderall, VyVanse, Concerta or naturally stimulant substances such as ginseng, green tea, rhodiola and L-tyrosine (an amino acid). Apart from these, ample physical exercise helps increase the levels of dopamine. Similarly, regular supplements of fish oil also help increase the levels of dopamine in the brain.

- **Inattentive ADHD:**

THIS TYPE OF ADHD RESPONDS WELL TO TREATMENT. IN fact, complete remission is seen in most patients provided he is treated properly. The goal here is to increase the levels of dopamine, similar to the previous treatment. Regular supplements of L-tyrosine help synthesize dopamine and are especially effective when taken on an empty stomach. Other stimulants like Adderall, Vyvanse or Concerta may be taken to alleviate symptoms. A low carbohydrate, high protein diet and a regular exercise regime helps achieve the desired results much faster.

• Over-Focused ADHD:

SINCE THIS PARTICULAR SUBTYPE IS ASSOCIATED WITH LOW serotonin and dopamine both, the aim is to restore the levels of both these chemicals in the brain. Stimulant medicines are not very effective in this type, rather they adversely make the person even more anxious and worried. Medicines like Effexor, Pristique and Cymbalta are helpful in increasing both dopamine and serotonin levels. High protein diets are to be avoided here as well.

• Temporal Lobe ADHD

THE MOST PREDOMINANT NEUROTRANSMITTER IN THIS PART of the brain is gamma aminobutyric acid, also known as GABA. Therefore this chemical is administered to help prevent brain cells from giving out excessive signals. Magnesium supplements help decrease anxiety and irritability in this particular condition. The mood swings have been successfully managed in some patients by taking anticonvulsants. Some of the more organic treatments include gingko or vincopocetine, which are particularly helpful in reversing learning and memory problems.

• Limbic ADHD:

THE TREATMENT RECOMMENDED HERE INCLUDES DL-phenylalanine, L-tyrosine and s-adenosyl-methionine. The medicine which has shown much promise is Wellbutrin. This is probably because it increases the levels of dopamine in the brain. Another effective option is Imipramine. As mentioned before, medication coupled with exercise, regular fish oil supplements and the appropriate diet will be able to reverse the disabilities much faster.

• Ring of Fire ADHD:

THIS SUBTYPE STANDS OUT FROM OTHER BECAUSE OF THE excessive activity seen in the brain. GABA and Serotonin medications are taken to boost their levels and a strict diet regimen is followed in the case of possible allergy being the exacerbating factor. Other medications include 5HTP and L-Tyrosine supplements and anticonvulsants. Overall hyperactivity can be curbed by administering guanfacine and clonidine.

• Anxious ADHD

THE GOAL OF TREATMENT HERE IS TO INCREASE THE LEVELS of GABA and dopamine levels. The stimulants are not advised to be taken alone otherwise they cause further anxiety in the patient. Certain calming substances include L-theonine, relora, holy basil and magnesium. Sometimes, the clinician may have to resort to tricyclic antidepressants in order to lower the levels of anxiety. The symptoms of prefrontal cortex can easily be calmed by neurofeedback.

INSIDE YOUR CHILD'S MIND

※

I t is very easy to observe an ADHD child and immediately point out what's wrong with him. That's because our minds immediately identify what they are doing wrong. But, ADHD minds, on the other hand, don't register what action is appropriate or inappropriate. Even if the mind does recognize something is wrong, it refuses to give in. You feel frustrated that your child is out of your control and doesn't listen to you. ADHD children feel the same way. Their minds are not under their control.

The normal mind has an automatic filter mechanism whereby it can *choose* to absorb certain types of information while redirecting other sorts of information. The ADHD mind, on the other hand, takes in *everything*. Not only this but these people are unable to sort out this information priority wise and almost everything seems to be 'important'. This inevitably results in them holding onto the information which is not as important the one that they didn't register properly. In the words of one sufferer, it is as if there are thousands of television screens in front of you and all your mind does is try and look at all of them the same time, jumping from one screen to another. This can be overcome by separating tasks and focusing on task at a time.

As mentioned before, one of the core symptoms of this disorder is *overstimulation*. The stimuli build up quickly and tend to accumulate to the extent that the person becomes frustrated. This frustration can be channeled outward as in extroverts who throw fits and become aggressive, or it may be kept in by introverts who ten to become anxious, upset and extremely edgy. This needs to take care of by clearing the mind, much like a reset button. This 'button' is different for everyone. What helps is taking a break and sitting in solitude for a couple of minutes. Children usually achieve their calm by fidgeting with their hands and feet or squirming in their seats.

One of the main issues encountered by people affected by ADHD is retrieving and accessing short term and long term memory. This is a source of immense frustration for patients. The fact that they experience difficulty in remembering things shows in their impulsivity and tendency to answer 'out of turn'. This is because they feel as if they don't answer immediately they will forget the answer and will never be able to answer. Another feature that this symptom brings out is that people affected by ADHD tend to hold on to certain items, both big and small, just so they don't forget the memories associated with those items. Children with ADHD can be encouraged to remember things via checklists, sticky notes, text messages or emails. Memories can be reinforced by maintaining scrap books with pictures and captions.

The reason why it is necessary to think from 'inside the mind' of a person with ADHD is because the hyper activity that is so often mentioned comes from within rather than being overtly expressed. The time period for which they get into the 'ADHD zone' is one in which the person is *free* from all of the said symptoms. One can get into the 'zone' about four or five times a day. During this time the person is not much different from an unaffected person. This waxing and waning of symptoms is what can be called the hallmark of ADHD; the symptoms can appear and reappear throughout one's life. A typical trigger for getting into the symptom free zone is by initiating something that is of interest to the person. In other words, people with ADHD have a license to do exactly what they *like* to do. Other situations responsible for getting people with ADHD into the zone include a challenging or competitive situation or an altogether new task. This is the reason behind the procrastinating behavior of people with ADHD; they simply cannot concentrate until it gets *interesting or challenging* enough for them to concentrate.

The reason ADHD people are set apart from non-ADHD people is because unaffected people have a completely different functioning of the nervous system. These people are also called 'neurotypical'. They pre-emptively decide what they have to do, how to get started on it and how to stick to it until the work has been completed. The decision making power and ability to focus on a task in these people is preceded by three main factors:

1. The concept of importance of the task in their minds,
2. The concept of secondary importance of the task, i.e. importance in *other* people's minds such as parents or teachers and
3. The concept of reward for finishing the task and punishment for not completing it.

The difference between an ADHD mind and a neurotypical mind comes in when the person with ADHD is unable to imply these concepts to initiate a task. Although they well understand the importance, like rewards and want to avoid punishment much like neurotypical people, they are unable to *imply* these concepts.

It is this inability to be motivated enough to complete tasks that can become crippling for ADHD affecting children in their adult lives. They will be unable to make major life decisions.

These differences between the minds of neurotypical and ADHD people are what create a rift between these two types of people. What is simple logic to one person, simply does not make sense to the other person. This is why education systems developed for neurotypical children will not work for children with ADHD; why they do not fit in a standard school system which seems to be working just fine for everyone else; why people with ADHD are inconsistent and unsuccessful with jobs that others tend to do well because the work is based on the concepts of *importance* an *rewards;* why ADHD people are disorganized because *organization* per se is based upon time management and prioritization and this is something ADHD people aren't very good at and this is why the person with ADHD seems confusing in indecisive because his mind simply won't let him *choose* a single option.

However unsure people with ADHD are about options, they are sure about one thing: their supernatural ability to concentrate and complete a task once they get engaged with it. Therefore the simple conclusion one can draw from this is that the problem does not lie with their nervous systems, it lies with the neurotypical instructions they are given from the time they were born.

ADHD AND FOODS

❧❧❧

W HAT TO EAT

By NOW YOU HAVE MOST LIKELY UNDERSTOOD THE CONCEPT that the treatment of ADHD isn't simply about administering medications but also about altering the child's lifestyle and diet, as well as engaging him in various activities. This chapter will be focused solely on the type of diet recommended for children with ADHD. This is not to say that an altered diet will be sufficient to reverse all ADHD symptoms. There are studies which have shown that certain symptoms of ADHD can be affected by what your child eats.

According to the latest guidelines put forward by the US Department of Agriculture, one half of the plate for *each* meal should consist of fruits and vegetables, one quarter should consist of carbohydrate and one half should consist of protein. This should be accompanied by some dairy of calcium rich food item. According to these guidelines, the important points to be noted are:

- Vegetables, fruits, whole grains and dairy products
- The source of carbohydrate should be *whole* grains rather than *processed*
- The main sources of protein should be poultry, lean meats, fish, eggs, nuts and beans
- Oil is essential for health and must ideally be derived from fish, nuts and liquid oils
- Foods containing saturated and trans fats, salt, cholesterol and added sugars should be avoided as far as possible

ANOTHER GUIDELINE THAT SHOULD BE FOLLOWED WHEN eating is that put forward by the Food and Nutrition Board; this is the Recommended Daily Allowance (RDA) of all macro and micro nutrients according to each age group. The simple definition of RDA of a specific nutrient is that which fulfills the requirement of more than 97% of the population. Ensuring that an ADHD child eats according to these recommendations is sure to help them.

Due to extensive research being conducted in the field of ADHD, it has been found that a diet high in saturated fats, refined sugars and salt, in short a typically *Western* diet, is associated with twice the incidence of ADHD as opposed to those who eat a healthier diet including omega-3 fatty acids, fiber and folic acid and low in fats and refined sugar.

PROTEINS AND CARBOHYDRATES
Proteins are macromolecules made up from smaller and

less complex molecules called amino acids. Foods rich in proteins are meats, fish, eggs, beans, nuts, seeds and dairy products. Proteins are the building blocks of cells and enzymes in the human body. Amino acids in their simpler forms are integral components of neurotransmitters in the brain. Glucose is carbohydrate in its most simple form and is the only form of nutrition accepted by the brain. Starches and carbohydrates on the other hand are the main source of energy for our bodies.

Children who have a substantial and filling breakfast are found to be more in control of their concentration and can focus on a task for a longer period of time than a child who has eaten very little or no breakfast. Proteins, specifically, are found to play a major role concentration control. Therefore a balanced breakfast with high protein as well as carbohydrate is the solution for ADHD children who wish to maintain a good level of concentration and cognitive performance over a long period of time. In another study, the effects of high blood sugar levels have little effect on the study performance of children, in fact high sugar foods and drink tend to improve symptoms of memory, attention, reaction time and mood. These beneficial effects are specifically seen when the blood sugar levels are rising.

Therefore, it is say safe to say that in order to achieve the best overall cognitive effects for a good five to six hours, one must have either a protein rich breakfast, or a balanced protein carbohydrate breakfast. Although we mentioned above that high sugar levels are associated with better performance, this improvement is rather short lived. Apart from being short lived, once the levels begin to recede, they actually plummet down much lower than before and the affected person may border on hypoglycemia. Such a situation will naturally aggravate any symptoms in inattentiveness and aggressiveness that a child may be predisposed to developing.

Needless to say these foods are a health hazard also because they disturb the mechanism responsible for taking glucose into the cell and predispose the child to developing diabetes. This is why carbohydrates which provide a sugar rush, like refined and processed carbohydrates should be avoided and, instead, unrefined carbohydrates should be preferred. Whole grains and barley are such examples; they are said to have a low glycemic index, which means that they release their nutrients slowly into the blood stream and there is no sugar rush that follows.

Now that we have established the importance of protein rich foods and unrefined carbohydrates for children with ADHD, we need to determine the amounts of both these nutrients that a child should take daily. The recommended daily allowance of protein is forty grams per day. They should ideally be consumed slowly throughout the day by taking about ten grams in each meal and about five grams per snack if the child is taking two snacks a day. Calculating the amount of protein in each food can be made easy by rough estimation. For instance, a sausage, an egg and a cup of yoghurt, all have around seven grams of proteins.

One way of reinforcing these studies and ensuring that this diet is effective for *your* child is to do a small experiment. During school holidays, give your child a protein rich breakfast one day, this should ideally include eggs, milk, meat and cheese. No cereal, fruits or juices. Observe your child's behavior that day and try and asses his cognitive and concentration abilities by giving him a task or puzzles to solve. On the very next day, give your child a low protein, high carbohydrate breakfast. This should consist purely of pancakes, waffles, syrup and fruits. Be sure to cut out on milk and meat on this day. Then, observe and test your child again.

You are sure to end up with results that reinforce the theory we have presented above. However, this does not mean that an ADHD child should always be ona high protein diet. Carbohydrates are absolutely essential for immediate energy and should be present in ample amounts in all meals. Nevertheless, breakfast should contain a relatively higher content of protein.

VITAMINS AND MINERALS

Vitamins and minerals are those substances which are required in very small amounts yet are extremely important for chemical reactions occurring in the body. Studies have shown that the levels of certain nutrients are directly associated with ADHD and its manifestations. These vitamins and minerals include iron, magnesium, zinc and polyunsaturated fatty acids. When regular supplements of these nutrients are given to children with ADHD, certain symptoms related to mood, cognition and behavior are seen to improve. However, these children were deficient in these nutrients to begin with, so it is difficult to say that whether they will be as effective when supplemented in children who have sufficient levels.

This aspect of nutrition is slightly difficult to challenge because of the extremely small amounts of each that are required. Also, when taken as supplements, all of the nutrients are not absorbed and are mostly excreted out in urine. Therefore, in a child who is eating a balanced diet as it is, it is wise to given him multi-vitamin and multi-mineral supplements containing half the recommended daily allowance, so that these nutrient levels actually *supplement* the levels achieved by normal diet and are as effective. Of course, if the child has a poor and misbalanced diet, then he should be given supplements containing the recommended daily allowance!

A multivitamin supplement is rich in vitamin A (retinoic acid). B1 (thiamine), B2 (niacin), B3 (riboflavin), B5 (pantothenic acid), B6 (pyridoxine), B12 (cyanocobalamin), C, D, E and zinc, manganese, copper, calcium and magnesium supplements. Certain other micronutrients like biotin, vitamin K, iodine, choline, selenium, inositol, antioxidants and other nutrients are also present. These nutrients are also present in fortified bread and milk. So that is also a good method of ensuring a balanced diet in children.

One important point to be noted about taking vitamin supplements is that certain vitamins are soluble and instead of being stored in the body they are excreted out in the urine. Other vitamins, which are fat soluble, such as vitamins A, D, E and K are stored in the body's fat content. Therefore, an excess of *these* vitamins is harmful and has potential side effects. Toxic levels of these vitamins can impair liver function and the central nervous system. Also, since ADHD children are on a host of other medications, they should consult with their doctors before starting supplements of any sort.

OMEGA-3 AND OMEGA-6 POLYUNSATURATED FATTY ACIDS

Despite the common notion that fatty acids are bad for health, these substance are integral for the normal functioning of our bodies. Fatty acids particularly have important roles in the central nervous, immune and endocrine systems. Some fatty acids are called *essential* fatty acids because they cannot be synthesized within the body like other substances and have to be taken in from external sources. Omega-3 fatty acids are found in algae, walnuts, leafy greens and salmon. They are also found in ample quantities in flax seeds, hemp seeds, sunflower seeds and chia seeds. Omega-6 fatty acids are found in meat, dairy, eggs and other vegetable oils. The ideal ratio of omega-3 to omega-6 that should be taken is a ratio of 4:1, omega-6 to omega-3fatty acids. However, the typical American diet consists of a ratio of about 20:1, omega-6 to omega-3 fatty acids. Thus, most of the American population is clearly deficient in omega-3 fatty acids.

The reason why omega-3s, also known as docosahexaenoic acid (DHA) and eicosapentaaenoic acid (EPA), and omega-6s fatty acids, also known as gamma-linoleic acid (GLA), are so *essential* for children with ADHD, is because they play very important roles in brain function. Children with ADHD reportedly have lower amounts of these fatty acids in their brains compared to children who don't have ADHD. Although studies conducted by giving solely omega-3 or omega-6 fatty acids have not yielded noticeable results, a combination of both omega-3 an domega-6 fatty acids, with a predominance of EPA, have shown favorable results. Certain foods containing ample EPA and DHA are fish, whereas those with high levels of GLA include evening primrose oil and borage oil.

The recommended allowance of omega-3 fatty acids is between 700-1600 mg per day for children and young adults. The recommended allowance of omega-6 GLA is 50 mg. Regular supplements must be taken for at least three to four months so as to replete the deficiencies that were present. Also, the symptoms that are controlled with these supplements have more to do with mood and anxiety rather than with inattentiveness, hyperactivity and other core symptoms of ADHD.

In any case, overdose should be avoided. The positive and negative effects seen after starting a new supplement must be scrutinized as every child has a different level of response.

WHAT *NOT* TO EAT

AS MENTIONED BEFORE, CERTAIN FOODS TEND TO HAVE AN adverse effect on children with ADHD. Their symptoms are aggravated and their performance is worsened. There are two strategies that are followed in order to eliminate these foods from the diet of an ADHD child. These strategies include the **Feingold Program** and simple **elimination of specific foods**.

The Feingold program is all about eliminating every type of artificial color and flavor that a child could possibly eat. These artificial substances are high in preservatives and salicylates. Therefore, all artificial colors, artificial flavors, preservatives including butylated hydroxytoluene (BHT), butylated hydoxyanisole (BHA), tertiary butylhydroxyquinone (TBHQ), aspirin, other non-steroidala nti inflammatory medicines, synthetic sweeteners, and other salicylates occurring naturally are eliminated from the diet for a minimum of six weeks. Foods containing high levels of natural salicylates include oranges, tangerines, apples, raisins, grapes, clementines, nectarines, peaches, currants, prunes, apricots, plums, cherries, berries, tomatoes, cucumbers, bell peppers, chilies, almonds, cloves, rose hips, paprika, apple cider vinegar, tea and coffee. Certain foods from this family are allowed, for instance pineapple, melons, banana, lemons, grapefruits, limes, mangoes, passionfruit, papaya and guava. Other allowed foods are fresh vegetables, nuts, spices, seeds, oils, meat, dairy products and whole grains.

Once this diet is being strictly followed and a consequent improvement is noticed, then the foods containing natural salicylates are added back one by one and observed for any adverse symptoms. However, if despite the elimination of these substances an improvement is not seen, then other sources of artificial substances must be looked for that are being unknowingly ingested, inhaled or used by the child.

The benefits of this sort of elimination diet are that children report an improvement in flexibility or adaptability, improved quality of sleep and certain other ADHD symptoms.

TIPS FOR PARENTS

❦

I f you think your child could possibly have ADHD or if your child has been recently diagnosed with ADHD, then you are sure to think of yourself as being between a rock and a hard place. Although challenging, dealing with this disorder is not entirely impossible. The earlier you embrace this condition and try overcoming it, the more motivated you child will be in combatting it. Here is a list of tips which might help you deal with your child:

- Be sure to *point out your child's mistakes* but convince him that it's okay as long as he's trying.
- *Eliminate all sources of distraction* when your teen is driving
- When you catch your child telling a lie, *give him another chance* to speak again so he may be tempted to tell you the truth
- Try giving your child *long acting medications* to overcome even the minor difficulties he feels he is facing
- Encourage your child to *get attached to a pet,*

preferably a dog. Dogs can prove to be the best companion to ADHD children when they misunderstood by everyone around them

- Urge your child to *speak out his emotions and feelings* when he feels strung up rather than silently act on them
- *Girls with ADHD* often tend to fly under the radar and must be observed further it they spend hours fidgeting or daydreaming
- Encourage your child to participate in *yoga, taek won do and gymnastics* as these activities tend to boost focus
- Break your child's over focus on video games by *lightly tapping* him on the shoulder and reminding him to get back to books
- If your child is having difficulty with some symptoms, like being unable to fall asleep, *don't blame yourself.* You being more stressed is not going to help unwind the stress in your child
- When your child is upset about the medication side effects of other difficulties he is facing, remind him of all the *strengths and positive qualities* he possesses.
- Use a *calendar* to manage and monitor your child's symptoms
- *Don't feel guilty* for wishing you didn't have this child, it's a perfectly normal reaction by ADHD parents. After all, you *are* human!
- Try and avoid the pressure from getting on your nerves by getting someone else to do the chores you *really* hate.
- Get your child to spend at least ten minutes a day on *mind-training apps* like Lumosity and Elevate. This will help develop focus and attentiveness.

- More than half the children with ADHD have inherited it. Embrace this possibility and try and figure out *whether you have it as well.*
- *Wake up half an hour earlier* to mentally prepare yourself for the day
- *Be vocal with love and appreciation* for your spouse, this makes children feel secure and happy.
- Take out time and *go to the gym* regularly. Exercise is as good an antidepressant as any medication.
- When scolding your child, remember how you felt while being scolded and try and *go easy on them.*
- If your child is a picky eater, don't force him to eat. Instead try and *supplement his diet.*
- Encourage *extracurricular activities* for your child, this helps them become more confident as well as become more social
- Once a tantrum has begun, get ready to leave the party so as to *avoid further aggravation* and not exhaust other people
- A *good high protein breakfast* option is plain yoghurt with fresh fruit. This will boost concentration all day long
- Curb a temper tantrum by giving your child *focused task* to engage his mind.
- Always take your children along when calling on someone so as to teach them how to *communicate with body language* and expressions
- Dedicate at least fifteen minutes a day to just listening to your ADHD child. Remember to *just* listen and not criticize
- ADHD is simply a *genetic biological disorder.* It's not anybody's fault!
- The more your child will *exercise* throughout the

day, the more exhausted he will be and the better he will sleep at night.

- Before reprimanding your child, make sure you *explain to him* what he's doing wrong before punishing him.
- Try *coinciding mealtimes* with your child's appetite bursts.
- How to be a good disciplinarian? Be *calm, specific, brief and consistent.*
- Always *create a checklist* for your child so he knows *exactly* what is expected of him
- Try and arrange for your child to *play with younger children*. This helps boost their self-confidence.
- *Don't undermine your importance* by not following out with the consequences you have already stated.
- If your child has a tendency to lose important papers, notices and reports? If yes then maybe he has *Executive Function Disorder.*
- A good way to deal with a possible outburst is to keep *balloons in your bag* and ask your child to inflate it when he feels like he is about to burst.
- *Encourage tennis* because this helps the child follow instructions and perform on an individual basis.
- A good way of helping your child concentrate is my making him *chew on gum or squeeze a small rubber ball* during long tests.
- Remember that most ADHD children are *hypersensitive*. Spanking them may be an emotional blow to them
- *Don't fool yourself* into thinking that you can calm your child down by reassurance, logic or lectures
- Teach your child how to be *responsible* by writing out instructions and illustrating with pictures

- *Punishing* your child for lying may make things worse.
- Make sure there is at least *an hour of silence* before bedtime, so that your child sleeps well
- Children who *exercise regularly* are better able to control their anger and aggressiveness.
- The minimum time that stimulant medicines take to act is an *hour* as they need this time to cross the blood brain barrier.
- *Fidgeting* intentionally helps control symptoms of anxiety.
- *Avoid negative comments* like 'why do u always oversleep', rather rephrase yourself with something like 'let's try waking up earlier tomorrow!'
- An optimal dose of medication is *not harmful* for a child's height or weight
- Define *goals which can be easily attained* and then reward your child for achieving those goals until they become a part of his routine behavior.

CLASSROOM TIPS

✿

Children often look up to their teachers more than their parents. Half of a child's development takes place in the classroom. Teachers have to take a different approach while dealing with children who have ADHD because their minds work differently. This is why dealing with them in the same manner as one deals with neuro typical children is an injustice. We have compiled a list of tips for teachers and students so as to improve the overall performance and grades of children who are affected by ADHD.

TIPS FOR PRESCHOOL AND PRIMARY SCHOOL TEACHERS

- Teaching these kids should include *problem based* and *student based* learning.
- Incorporate *music* and *dance* into classroom lessons. This is always helpful in memorizing facts and figures and it's a welcome getaway from the sober and serious classroom environment.
- Make sure a strict schedule is followed. Activities

and instructions must be announced before they begin.

- Be careful while choosing *punishments*. The one's like making the student stay back during recess affects the morale and concentration and may make things worse.
- Avoid changing routines too often; these children are comfortable with a situation when it becomes familiar. Don't hesitate to *repeat* study routines.
- Make sure the child with ADHD sits *near your desk* at the front of the classroom.
- Try and always *reward* children for small achievements, this will help other children work harder and keep their focus on the reward.
- *Avoid distractions* as much as possible. The window and the door are the two main sources of distraction in any classroom. Children with ADHD should be seated as far as possible from the windows and doors of the classroom.
- *Don't lose your patience*. These children have to fight with their minds to obey you. Go easy on them.
- Try and utilize *multiple intelligence* strategies into your teaching schedule. This helps stimulate other regions of the brain. The nine main intelligences that must be appealed to are naturalist, musical, logical-mathematical, existential, interpersonal, bodily kinesthetic, linguistic, intra-personal and spatial intelligence.
- *Keep in touch* with the child's parents. Know what strategies work for and against the child.
- Write down *clear, concise and specific directions*. When introducing a new activity, make sure the whole class in attentive.
- Try and *praise* the child for every answer given

correct. Avoid ridiculing him over wrong or incomplete answers.

- Use *pictures, figures, acronyms and colors* to help these children remember what you're teaching.
- Make sure the children are being given *brain breaks* after exhausting exercises.

TIPS FOR HIGH SCHOOL AND COLLEGE TEACHERS

- *Break down* large exercises in to smaller ones.
- Always provide the student with an *example or a model* as a standard.
- Help the child with *time management*. This is one of the most challenging tasks a person with ADHD has to face.
- Use *proactive* strategies with the student. Encourage him to speak up rather than prompting him.
- Give the student *sufficient breaks* to gather his thoughts together and focus on the task at hand.
- In case the child is misbehaving in school, use *pre decided and confidential cues* to correct him or reprimand him.
- Make sure the students who need the most help are *seated right at the front* of the class.
- Discuss or *model a situation* of possible outburst and advise the child how to curb his emotions in such a situation.
- *Role play* various social situations and make the child or teen practice his behavior in such situations.

- Provide as many *social* situations to such students as possible, this helps bring out the best in them.
- Once these children achieve something, be it good grades or even a minor challenge, be sure to appreciate and *positively reinforce* him.
- Provide opportunities and situations to such children so that they may *showcase their abilities* in front of other people. This helps build up their self-esteem and confidence.
- Give the students a *definite purpose* behind every activity they perform.
- Encourage the child to *appreciate himself* and his strengths rather than beat himself up about certain weakness.
- Give oral and visual instructions so that you appeal to all his senses and ensure that he understands the assignment that he has to complete. Also ask him to explain what he has understood of the instructions.

TIPS FOR STUDENTS

- Memorize information by drawing *pictures and diagrams*. This helps appeal to other areas of the brain and helps retain information for longer.
- Make *mnemonics* for everything. This is an excellent trick for memorizing facts.
- Create *whole sentences or acrostics* when trying to understand a concept.
- Use music and rhythm while studying to stimulate

the right side of the brain and hence bring more brain cells into use.

- Be sure to *pay attention* in class and ask the teacher questions in every session.
- *Make a list* of all the information that you remember after the class is over
- Stay on top of your *homework*. Studying over extended time periods rather than the night before will help you retain information in your long term memory.
- Advocate for yourself. If you feel you need a calculator, *ask for it*. If you feel you need extra time, ask for it. If you feel the general classroom is too distracting, ask for a separate quiet room to give your test in. Your mind works differently from others and so you have to treat it differently.
- Make sure you get *enough sleep*. Staying up late on an exam night is going to reduce your efficiency, if anything at all. Make it a point to go to bed early, even on weekends.
- Avoid taking junk food just before a test. The refined sugar will eventually cause hypoglycemia during the test and your brain won't function as well. Take *plain water and high protein snacks* instead. Foods such as meat, eggs and fish and rice are rich in choline, a substance which makes up an important neurotransmitter in the brain, this helps improve memory.
- You have a predisposition towards anxiety. Since this anxiety is going to get worse just before an exam, you need to take physical and mental measures to alleviate it. For instance, exercise, yoga or a simple brisk walk helps distress you. Mentally, you can visualize calming sceneries like a

waterfall or a rainforest. This should help you *calm down and be anxiety free.*

- If you find it difficult to sit in one place for too long, then take breaks. Be it a bathroom break, a break to go drink water or to go sharpen your pencil. Find an excuse and *just get up.*
- Once your exam is over, be sure to *reward yourself* for your hard work, regardless of how your paper went. The important point is that you worked hard.

DID YOU KNOW?

WE HAVE COMPILED CERTAIN FACTS AND QUOTES ABOUT ADHD that most of the general public is unaware about. The reason why we feel this is an important addition to this book is that when a loved one is suffering from this disorder, you can never have enough knowledge about it. Every little piece of information counts and is sure to help you cope with this disorder just a little bit better than before. Every success story is an inspiration. For instance, did you know:

- IQ and ADHD are completely independent of one another and children with ADHD usually have average or above average IQ levels?
- There no single gene or parent responsible for ADHD. The cause of the disorder is complex and multifactorial.
- ADHD cases have been reported as far back as 1902.
- Over focusing on a certain task for several hours is a symptom present in one of the subtypes of

ADHD and is an incredible ability which may help the child achieve better grades than his peers.

- A strong will power is medicine enough to cure even the most severe form of ADHD.
- Tim Howard, superstar of the world cup 2014 was diagnosed with ADHD, Obsessive Compulsive disorder and Tourette's syndrome at the age of 11 years.
- 'The ADHD brain is a Ferrari engine, with the brakes of a bicycle'

- Dr. Ned Hallowell

- ADHD children have the outstanding ability to think outside the box and come up with creative ideas like Apple, Instagram and Tesla.
- The constant fidgeting of ADHD children is good for them in the way that it helps them overcome their anxiety and helps them focus.
- Daydreaming is simply a prelude to a master idea and creativity.
- 'Some people have a negative attitude, and *that's* their only disability'

-Marla Runyan

- The three adjectives mostly used for ADHD children by their friends are: *generous, compassionate and empathetic.*
- Some people with a history of ADHD have played pivotal roles in changing the world. These include Sir Richard Branson, Ingvar Kamprad (founder of Ikea) and JetBlue's David Neelman.
- The rhythm of music has a soothing and calming

effect on the ADHD mind which is then able to focus better.

- The ADHD brain is a finely tuned but extremely rare orchestra where the conductor is trying to lead 12 songs simultaneously.
- Teachers who implement visual, tactile and audio learning strategies in children are able to make a tremendous difference in the development and learning of their students.
- 'Whoever put deficit and disorder into ADHD? Labelling the weaknesses of children rather than their strengths is extremely counterproductive!

-Alison Larkin

- Certain natural methods of calming and training the ADHD mind include martial arts like taek won do and tai chin.
- The ADHD brain is not defective or slow, it is a perfectly normal nervous system which functions just fine and follows its own set of unique rules.
- ADHD is usually hereditary, rather than being treated as a curse it should be considered a special bond between parent and child.
- 'Medicines alone are not enough. We can't only treat the neurochemical deficiency'

-Dr. Larry Silver

- An integral aspect of treatment for ADHD is relaxation, so take this luxury as an absolute necessity for you and go get that massage!
- Micheal Phelp's school teacher was always complaining of his lack of self-discipline and focus;

he went on to win 18 Olympic Gold medals, a
world record.

Therefore you can rest assured that being diagnosed with
ADHD is not the end of the world. It is a perfectly treatable
condition and may sometimes even enable the person
affected to achieve great things!

Afterword

Having read all the information above, you must have realized that ADHD is *not a disease*, in fact it's not even a *disorder* as it is often referred to. It's simply something that makes your child different from a lot of other children. In some cases they are smarter and more genius than the other children, also referred to as neurotypical children. Not being *typical* is not necessarily a bad thing. Take it as a challenge. If you also suffer from ADHD then you should be thankful that you are in a position to understand your child better. In any case, you have to realize one thing: how your child deals with his condition; how well he does in school; to what extent he overcomes his weakness, all depends upon *you!*

Make him feel important rather than different or difficult; help him develop his self-esteem and confidence; perhaps he might grow up to another Michael Phelps, you never know. Instead of being overwhelmed by the fact that your child has a *disorder*, be grateful that he doesn't have a terminal illness, as many American children today do. We want you to help yourself and help your child, and that is precisely why this short e-book has been written. So read it; make your child read it; and get ready to conquer the condition that is ADHD.